53 Stress Reduction Meal Recipes to Help You Get Through Tough Times and Moments of Anxiety:

Delicious Meal Recipes to Help You Cope With Stress

By

Joe Correa CSN

COPYRIGHT

© 2016 Live Stronger Faster Inc.

This publication is designed to provide accurate and authoritative information in regard to the subject matter covered. It is sold with the understanding that neither the author nor the publisher is engaged in rendering medical advice. If medical advice or assistance is needed, consult with a doctor. This book is considered a guide and should not be used in any way detrimental to your health. Consult with a physician before starting this nutritional plan to make sure it's right for you.

ACKNOWLEDGEMENTS

This book is dedicated to my friends and family that have had mild or serious illnesses so that you may find a solution and make the necessary changes in your life.

53 Stress Reduction Meal Recipes to Help You Get Through Tough Times and Moments of Anxiety:

Delicious Meal Recipes to Help You Cope With Stress

By

Joe Correa CSN

CONTENTS

ABOUT THE AUTHOR

After years of Research, I honestly believe in the positive effects that proper nutrition can have over the body and mind. My knowledge and experience has helped me live healthier throughout the years and which I have shared with family and friends. The more you know about eating and drinking healthier, the sooner you will want to change your life and eating habits.

Nutrition is a key part in the process of being healthy and living longer so get started today. The first step is the most important and the most significant.

INTRODUCTION

53 Stress Reduction Meal Recipes to Help You Get Through Tough Times and Moments of Anxiety: Delicious Meal Recipes to Help You Cope With Stress

By Joe Correa CSN

Stress is an emotional condition that is common for all human beings. There isn't a single person in this world who hasn't felt stressed-out at some point in life. Stress is often correlated to binge eating which occurs as some form of response to stressful situations.

We can't define stress as a disease, but more like an emotional state and the feeling of being unable to handle our problems. It slowly, without even noticing it, starts affecting our health in so many different ways. Our immune system starts to weaken, we feel tired, sick, and without energy. This leads our body into a state of a hormonal disbalance and sugar levels drop, which often results in overeating. Stress is a proven trigger to so many different and way more dangerous diseases. It's one of the leading causes of heart diseases, having strokes, different organ failures, hormonal imbalance and everything related to it, etc. Binge eating, as a final product of stress, leads to becoming overweight and many other problems that go along with it. It is a vicious cycle that should be stopped and corrected as soon as possible.

Eliminating all the factors that cause stress is almost impossible. However, the best way to boost your energy and leave stress behind is starting a healthy diet! This is a no-brainer. A healthy diet will balance your entire body in a way that you can't even imagine. A balanced diet will stabilize your blood sugar levels and give you enough energy to deal with a stressful situation and emotional issues in the best possible manner.

This is exactly why I have created this book with healthy and great-tasting recipes that focus on increasing fiber and good carbs to keep blood sugar levels in check. These recipes are full of natural sources of all kinds of nutrients your body so desperately needs in order to deal with everyday's life. Fruits and vegetables, legumes, beans, healthy lean meats, lots of salmon and olive oil, nuts and seeds. There is absolutely nothing better than eating smarter to lower stress levels.

This book focuses on foods rich in vitamin C, vitamin B, and Magnesium.

Foods with ingredients like lemons, oranges, pepper, tomatoes, and leafy greens are a great natural source of vitamin C. This vitamin has a strong physical and psychological impact on people dealing with stress.

Vitamin B is an energy booster that will give you the mental and physical strength to recover after a stressful situation. Spinach, avocado, nuts, and fish, are just some of the ingredients that I have included in these recipes to increase this essential stress-management vitamin.

Magnesium is in charge of a muscle relaxation and anxiety management which is included in many of the foods in the recipes that appear in this book. You'll find some natural magnesium boosters like nuts, brown rice, and beans in different mouth-watering combinations.

A proper, balanced diet full of these precious nutrients helps not only deal with stress and binge eating but will affect your entire life and health.

Let this book serve as motivation for a more relaxing and stress-free life!

53 STRESS REDUCTION MEAL RECIPES TO HELP YOU GET THROUGH TOUGH TIMES AND MOMENTS OF ANXIETY: DELICIOUS MEAL RECIPES TO HELP YOU COPE WITH STRESS

1.   Kidney Bean Mushroom Stew

Ingredients:

4 cups of kidney beans, pre-cooked, drained

1 lb of button mushrooms, chopped

1 medium-sized onion, finely chopped

2 cups of tomatoes, diced

4 garlic cloves, minced

½ cup of fresh basil, minced

1 tbsp of dried thyme, ground

1 tsp of vegetable oil

2 tsp of fresh rosemary, finely chopped

½ tsp of salt

¼ tsp of black pepper, ground

Preparation:

Place the beans in a pot of boiling water and cook for 2 minutes. Set aside for 2 hours.

Preheat the oil in a large skillet over a medium-high temperature. Add onions and garlic and stir-fry for 10 minutes, until translucent.

Now, add tomatoes, mushrooms, thyme, basil, and rosemary.Cook for 10 minutes and stir in the beans. Add water to adjust thickness if needed. Reduce the heat to low and cover with a lid. Cook for 40 minutes and sprinkle with salt and pepper to taste. Remove from the heat and give it a good stir.

Serve warm.

Nutrition information per serving: Kcal: 346, Protein: 23.4g, Carbs: 62.3g, Fats: 1.9g

2.   Tomato Soup

Ingredients:

1 lb of tomatoes, diced

3 medium-sized bell peppers, diced

1 large carrot, sliced

3 garlic cloves, minced

1 large onion, chopped

2 tbsp of sour cream

½ cup of fresh basil, finely chopped

1 tsp of vegetable seasoning mix

¼ tsp of black pepper, ground

1 tsp of dried thyme, ground

¼ tsp of salt

Preparation:

Combine onion, garlic, and 2 tablespoons of water in a large nonstick skillet over a medium-high temperature. Cook for about 3-4 minutes or until water evaporates.

Add bell peppers, carrot and ½ cup of water. Cook until fork-tender. Add tomatoes, basil, dried thyme and stir well to combine. Reduce the heat to low and cover with a lid. Cook for 20 minutes and remove from the heat. Transfer the mixture to a food processor and blend until smooth. Return mixture to the skillet. Heat it up sprinkle with salt and pepper.

Serve warm.

Nutrition information per serving: Kcal: 178, Protein: 5.9g, Carbs: 35.5g, Fats: 3.6g

3. Pasta with Arugula Sauce

Ingredients:

2 lbs of pasta, pre-cooked

2 cups of fresh arugula, trimmed

1 cup of cream cheese

2 tsp of lemon juice, freshly squeezed

4 garlic cloves, minced

2 tbsp of pine nuts, toasted

½ tsp of salt

Preparation:

Cook pasta using package instructions. Drain well and set aside.

Meanwhile, combine cheese, arugula, lemon juice, garlic, and salt in a food processor. Blend until nicely smooth. Pour the sauce over the pasta and top with pine nuts.

Serve.

Nutrition information per serving: Kcal: 595, Protein: 20.7g, Carbs: 85.1g, Fats: 19.0g

4.　　Salmon with Salsa Potatoes

Ingredients:

2 lbs of wild salmon filets, skinless and boneless

1 tbsp of olive oil

1 tbsp of rosemary, finely chopped

½ tsp of sea salt

4 small potatoes, peeled and chopped

For the salsa:

2 medium-sized tomatoes, diced

1 small onion, diced

¼ cup of fresh parsley, chopped

1 tbsp of lemon juice

1 tsp of apple cider vinegar

½ tsp of salt

Preparation:

Place the potatoes in a pot of boiling water. Cook until fork-tender. Remove from the heat and drain. Transfer to a serving plate and set aside.

Combine all salsa ingredients in a food processor and blend until smooth. Transfer to a bowl and set aside.

Preheat the oil on a large nonstick pan over a medium-high temperature. Add meat and cook for about 4-5 minutes, or until set. Transfer the meat to a serving plate with potatoes. Sprinkle the meat with rosemary and salt. Pour the salsa over the potatoes and serve.

Nutrition information per serving: Kcal: 235, Protein: 23.9g, Carbs: 15.8g, Fats: 9.0g

5.   Avocado Chutney

Ingredients:

2 large avocados, pitted, peeled, and chopped

1 medium-sized onion, diced

1 tsp of fresh ginger, grated

1 tsp of cumin, ground

½ cup of fresh mint, finely chopped

1 tbsp of olive oil

½ tsp of salt

¼ tsp of black pepper, ground

Preparation:

Preheat the oil in a large skillet over a medium-high temperature. Add onions and stir-fry until translucent. Stir in cumin and ginger and cook for about 3-4 minutes more. Remove the skillet from the heat and stir in avocado and mint.

Sprinkle with some salt and pepper to taste and serve.

Nutrition information per serving: Kcal: 340, Protein: 3.6g, Carbs: 17.1g, Fats: 31.2g

6.   Basmati Rice

Ingredients:

3 cups of basmati rice

2 small red onions, diced

1 cup of spring onions, chopped

1 large bell pepper, chopped

1 medium-sized carrot, chopped

3 tbsp of lemon juice

1 tbsp of balsamic vinegar

1 tsp of curry powder

½ tsp of Cayenne pepper, ground

½ tsp of salt

¼ tsp of black pepper, ground

Preparation:

Mix together lemon juice, vinegar, curry, Cayenne pepper, salt, and pepper in a mixing bowl. Set aside to allow flavors to mingle.

Place the rice in a deep pot. Pour 6 cups of water and bring it to a boil. Now, reduce the heat to low and cover with a lid. Cook for 40 minutes, or until tender. Remove from the heat and drain. Set aside.

Meanwhile, combine red onions, spring onions, and carrot in a large bowl. Drizzle with lemon juice mixture and stir well. Add rice and mix all to combine.

Serve.

Nutrition information per serving: Kcal: 440, Protein: 9.1g, Carbs: 96.4g, Fats: 1.0g

7.   Orange Beet Salad

Ingredients:

2 large oranges, peeled and wedged

5 medium-sized beets, trimmed, peeled

2 cups of Romaine lettuce, chopped

2 cups of black beans, pre-cooked

1 tbsp of red wine vinegar

3 tbsp of fresh dill, minced

2 tbsp of extra-virgin olive oil

2 tbsp of almonds, roughly chopped

½ tsp of salt

¼ tsp of black pepper, ground

Preparation:

Mix together vinegar, oil, dill, salt, and pepper in a mixing bowl. Set aside.

Place the beets in a deep pot and add water enough to cover it. Bring it to a boil then reduce the heat. Cover with a lid and cook for about 20-25 minutes, or until fork-tender. Remove from the heat and drain well. Set aside.

Meanwhile, place the beans in a pot of boiling water. Cook until soften, then remove and drain well. Set aside.

Now, combine beets, beans, and oranges in a large bowl. Drizzle with dressing and toss well to coat.

Place a handful of lettuce on a serving plate and spoon the beet salad. Top with almonds and sprinkle with salt and pepper, if needed.

Nutrition information per serving: Kcal: 345, Protein: 16.8g, Carbs: 57.8g, Fats: 6.9g

8.   Zucchini Cream Soup

Ingredients:

4 medium-sized zucchinis, peeled and chopped

1 medium-sized onion, chopped

2 cups of vegetable broth

1 cup of plain yogurt

1 tsp of dried thyme, minced

1 tsp of nutmeg

1 tsp of lime zest

½ tsp of black pepper, ground

½ tsp of salt

Preparation:

Combine onions and 2 tablespoons of water in a large nonstick skillet over a medium-high temperature. Add zucchinis and cook for 5 minutes stirring constantly. Pour the vegetable stock and stir in nutmeg, thyme, and lime zest.

Cook for another 15 minutes, or until fork-tender. Remove from the heat and transfer to a food processor.

Blend until nicely smooth, then return to the skillet. Stir in the yogurt and heat it up. Sprinkle with salt and pepper if needed and serve.

Nutrition information per serving: Kcal: 63, Protein: 5.0g, Carbs: 8.3g, Fats: 1.2g

9.   Cucumber Tuna Wraps

Ingredients:

4 cans of tuna, drained

2 medium-sized cucumbers, chopped

½ cup of shallots, finely chopped

4 tbsp of mayonnaise

¼ cup of lemon juice

2 tbsp of sour cream

½ tsp of salt

¼ tsp of black pepper, ground

1 large lettuce head

Preparation:

Mix together mayonnaise, lemon juice, sour cream, and a pinch of salt in a small bowl. Set aside.

Combine tuna, shallots, cucumber in a large bowl. Stir in the previously made mixture and toss to mix well with a spoon.

Spread the lettuce leaves on a serving plate and spoon the mixture. Wrap and secure with a toothpick. Serve immediately.

Nutrition information per serving: Kcal: 253, Protein: 28.1g, Carbs: 7.4g, Fats: 11.9g

10.   Vegetable Hash

Ingredients:

2 cups of white beans, pre-cooked

½ cup of leeks, finely chopped

1 large bell pepper, finely chopped

2 small potatoes, peeled and chopped

1 cup of fresh kale, chopped

2 garlic cloves, minced

2 tsp of fresh rosemary, finely chopped

2 tbsp of lemon juice

1 tbsp of lemon zest

1 tsp of salt

½ tsp of black pepper, ground

Preparation:

Place potatoes in a pot of boiling water. Cook until soften and remove from the heat. Drain well and set aside. Repeat the process with beans.

Combine leeks, pepper and 2 tablespoons of water in a large nonstick saucepan over a medium-high temperature. Cook for 2 minutes, then add garlic. Sprinkle with rosemary and stir well. Add potatoes, lemon juice, and beans. Cook for about 8-10 minutes then add kale. Cook for another 5 minutes, or until kale soften. Sprinkle with lemon zest, salt, and pepper before serving.

Nutrition information per serving: Kcal: 342, Protein: 21.0g, Carbs: 65.1g, Fats: 1.0g

11.   Gingerbread Cookies

Ingredients:

2 cups of whole-wheat flour

1 tsp of baking soda

1 tsp of ginger, ground

1 tsp of cinnamon, ground

½ cup of applesauce

2 tbsp of maple syrup

2 tbsp of fig jam

1 tsp of vanilla extract

Preparation:

Preheat the oven to 375°F.

Combine flour, baking soda, cinnamon, ginger, and vanilla. Stir well then add maple syrup, applesauce, and fig jam. Mix until you get a nice batter. Form the cookies in desired size or shape.

Place a baking paper over a large baking sheet. Spread the cookies with 2 inches of space in between. Bake for 5-6 minutes, or until crispy browned. Remove from the oven and let it cool for a while.

Serve with honey or milk. This is, however, optional.

Nutrition information per serving: Kcal: 91, Protein: 2.2g, Carbs: 19.6g, Fats: 0.2g

12.   Juicy Beef & Green Beans

Ingredients:

2 lbs of lean beef, cut into bite-sized pieces

2 large bell pepper, seeded and stripped

4 garlic cloves, minced

½ cup of fresh dill, finely chopped

2 cups of green beans, pre-cooked

3 tbsp of olive oil

1 tbsp of lemon juice

¼ tsp of Cayenne pepper, ground

½ tsp of salt

¼ tsp of black pepper, ground

Preparation:

Preheat the oven to 375°F.

Combine bell peppers, 2 tablespoons of oil, garlic, dill, lemon juice, cayenne pepper, salt, and pepper in a food processor. Blend until smooth and set aside.

Place the green beans in a pot of boiling water and cook until fork-tender. remove from the heat and drain well. Set aside.

Preheat the remaining oil in a large skillet over a medium-high temperature. Add meat and sprinkle with salt and pepper to taste. Cook for 10 minutes, or until golden brown. Remove from the heat and transfer to a serving plate with green beans. Drizzle with dressing and serve.

Nutrition information per serving: Kcal: 379, Protein: 47.9g, Carbs: 8.7g, Fats: 16.8g

13.   Cooked Red Cabbage and Apples

Ingredients:

1 large red cabbage head, shredded

2 medium-sized carrots, diced

1 cup of fresh celery, diced

2 medium-sized apples, peeled, cored and chopped

1 medium-sized onion, diced

2 tbsp of yellow mustard

4 tbsp of red wine vinegar

2 tbsp of olive oil

1 tsp of dried thyme, ground

½ tsp of salt

¼ tsp of black pepper, ground

Preparation:

Preheat the oil in a large nonstick skillet over a medium-high temperature. Add onions and stir-fry for a few minutes until translucent. Add celery, carrots, about 2 tablespoons of water, thyme, vinegar, and mustard. Cook for 5 minutes, stirring occasionally.

Add apples and cabbage and reduce the heat to low. Cover with a lid and cook for 20 minutes, or until tender.

Sprinkle with salt and pepper to taste before serving.

Nutrition information per serving: Kcal: 133, Protein: 2.5g, Carbs: 21.9g, Fats: 5.2g

14.   Oven-Baked Creamy Turkey Avocado

Ingredients:

4 lbs of turkey breasts, thinly sliced

1 medium-sized avocado, pitted, peeled, and chopped

1 large bell pepper, chopped

1 cup of Parmesan cheese, shredded

2 tbsp of fresh parsley, finely chopped

2 tbsp of Dijon mustard

½ cup of corn, kernel removed

4 tbsp of butter

½ tsp of Himalayan salt

Preparation:

Preheat the oven to 375°F.

Coat the meat with mustard in a large bowl. Set aside.

Melt the butter in a nonstick skillet over a medium-high temperature. Add avocado, pepper, cheese, parsley, and corn. Stir and cook until cheese is melted. Remove from the heat and transfer the mixture to a large baking dish. Add meat and coat with mixture. Cover the dish with aluminum foil and put it in the oven.

Bake for 45 minutes, or until heated trough. Remove from the oven and let it cool for a while before serving.

Nutrition information per serving: Kcal: 315, Protein: 35.1g, Carbs: 12.3g, Fats: 13.9g

15.   Garlic Meatballs

Ingredients:

1lb lean beef, minced

7 oz of white rice

2 small onions, peeled and finely chopped

2 garlic cloves, crushed

1 large egg, beaten

1 large potato, peeled and sliced

3 tbsp of extra-virgin olive oil

1 tsp of salt

Preparation:

In a large bowl, combine lean ground beef with rice, finely chopped onions, crushed garlic, one beaten egg, and salt. Shape the mixture into 15-20 meatballs, depending on the size.

Grease the bottom of your slow cooker with three tablespoons of olive oil. Make the first layer with sliced potatoes and top with meatballs.

Cover, set the heat to low and cook for 6-8 hours.

Nutrition information per serving: Kcal: 468, Protein: 33.4g, Carbs: 47.0g, Fats: 15.3g

16.   Peanut Butter Chicken

Ingredients:

4 lbs of chicken filets, thinly sliced

4 tbsp of peanut butter

1 cup of skim milk

¼ cup of fresh cilantro, finely chopped

4 tbsp of vegetable oil

4 tsp of ginger, ground

1 tbsp of sea salt

¼ tsp of black pepper, ground

Preparation:

Preheat the oven to 400°F.

Place the meat in a large baking dish and coat with sea salt. Set aside.

Preheat the oil in a large nonstick saucepan over a medium-high temperature. Add milk, cilantro, and ginger. Cook for 2 minutes then stir in ginger and pepper. Cook for another 2 minutes then add peanut butter. Stir well to combine and cook for another minute. Remove from the heat.

Pour the peanut butter mixture over the meat. Cover with a lid and place it in the oven. Bake for about 15-20 minutes, or until golden brown. Remove the lid and bake for 2 more minutes. Remove from the oven and let it cool for a while before serving.

Nutrition information per serving: Kcal: 371, Protein: 55.1g, Carbs: 3.0g, Fats: 14.2g

17.   Choco-Berry Smoothie

Ingredients:

1 cup of fresh strawberries

1 cup of frozen raspberries

5 egg whites

½ cup of coconut milk

¼ cup of chocolate chips

1 tbsp of honey

1 tbsp of flaxseed

Preparation:

Combine strawberries, raspberries, egg whites, coconut milk, and chocolate chips in a food processor. Blend until nicely smooth. Add water to adjust the thickness. Add honey and re-blend. Transfer the mixture to a serving glasses and top with flaxseeds for extra taste and nutrients.

Enjoy!

Nutrition information per serving: Kcal: 330, Protein: 9.3g, Carbs: 42.9g, Fats: 14.8g

18.   Toasted Nuts

Ingredients:

½ cup of almonds

½ cup of pistachios

½ cup of cashews

½ cup of walnuts

4 tbsp of butter

1 tsp of nutmeg

1 tsp of orange zest

1 tsp of cinnamon, ground

1 tsp of ginger, ground

1 tsp of salt

Preparation:

Preheat the oven to 350°F.

Combine all nuts in a large bowl.

Place some baking paper on a large baking dish and spread the nuts. Put it in the oven and roast for about 8-

10 minutes. Remove from the oven and set aside to cool for a while.

Melt the butter in a large nonstick frying pan over a medium-high temperature. Add cinnamon, nutmeg, ginger,salt, and orange zest. Stir well to combine and add nuts. Cook 1 minute and remove from the heat.

Serve immediately.

Nutrition information per serving: Kcal: 412, Protein: 10.6g, Carbs: 12.9g, Fats: 38.4g

19.   Creamy Lemon Salmon with Spinach

Ingredients:

2 lbs of wild salmon filets, thinly sliced

4 cups of spinach, finely chopped

1 cup of coconut milk

½ cup of lemon juice

1 tbsp of lemon zest

4 tbsp of fresh parsley, finely chopped

2 tbsp of pine nuts

2 tbsp of olive oil

1 tsp of salt

¼ tsp of black pepper, freshly ground

Preparation:

Preheat 1 tablespoon of oil in a large nonstick skillet over a medium-high temperature. Add meat and sprinkle with some salt to taste. Cook for 5 minutes on each side, or until golden brown. Set aside

Preheat the remaining oil in a separate frying pan and add spinach. Cook until slightly soften. Stir in pine nuts and cook for 1 minute more. Remove from the heat and transfer to a serving plate. Top with salmon and set aside.

Combine coconut milk and lemon juice in a medium saucepan. Heat it up and pour over the meat. Sprinkle with lemon zest before serving.

Nutrition information per serving: Kcal: 363, Protein: 31.5g, Carbs: 4.2g, Fats: 25.8g

20.   Chocolate Orange Yogurt

Ingredients:

1 cup of plain yogurt, or Greek yogurt

¼ cup of dark chocolate, grated

1 large orange, peeled and wedged

1 tbsp of honey

1 tbsp of chia seeds

A few mint leaves

Preparation:

Combine yogurt and chia in a medium bowl. Stir in the honey and mix well with a spoon.

Add grated chocolate and orange. Mix well and sprinkle with some fresh mint to taste.

Nutrition information per serving: Kcal: 268, Protein: 12.9g, Carbs: 36.0g, Fats: 9.6g

21.   Veal Steak in Garlic and Red Pepper Sauce

Ingredients:

1 lb of veal steak, boneless

3 large bell peppers, chopped

3 tbsp. of olive oil

4 cloves of garlic, chopped

1 small onion, chopped

1 tsp. of dried rosemary, finely chopped

½ cup of water

Non-fat cooking spray

Preparation:

Preheat oven to 350°F.

Lightly coat a baking sheet with cooking spray. Place the meat on a baking sheet and cook for 60 minutes.

Meanwhile, cut each pepper in half, remove the stem and seeds. Finely chop your peppers. Heat up the olive oil in a saucepan and add garlic and onion. Saute until translucent. This should take no more than 5 minutes. Stir constantly. Add peppers, rosemary and ½ cup of water (you can add some more water if the sauce is too thick). Bring it to a boil and reduce the heat to minimum. Cook for 10-15 minutes. Set aside.

When the meat is nice and tender, remove from the oven and transfer to a plate. Pour the pepper sauce over the meat chops and serve.

Nutrition information per serving: Kcal: 258, Protein: 46.0g, Carbs: 17.2g, Fats: 18.3g

22. Eggplant and Ground Beef Casserole

Ingredients:

2 large eggplants, thinly sliced

1 cup of lean beef, ground

1 medium-sized onion, chopped

1 tsp of olive oil

¼ tsp of black pepper, freshly ground

2 medium-sized tomatoes, cubed

3 tbsp of fresh parsley, finely chopped

Preparation:

Preheat the oven to 300°F.

Peel the eggplants and cut lengthwise into thin sheets. Put them in a bowl, and leave them to sit for at least an hour. Roll them in beaten eggs.

Preheat the oil in a large skillet over a medium-high temperature. Add eggplants and fry for 3 minutes on each side, or until set. Set aside.

Preheat the remaining oil in the same skillet. Stir-fry the onions until translucent, then add, tomato, and sprinkle with pepper and parsley. Cook for 2 minutes and add meat. Cook until tender.

Remove from the heat and set aside to cool for a while.

Combine meat and vegetable mixture and egg in an ovenproof dish and spread on the bottom. Make one layer with eggplants, then again meat and veggies. Repeat the process with remaining ingredients.

Bake for 30 minutes or until doneness. Remove from the oven and serve.

Nutrition information per serving: Kcal: 114, Protein: 14.2g, Carbs: 21.6g, Fats: 9.7g

23.   Coco Vanilla Smoothie

Ingredients:

1 cup of coconut milk

½ cup of water

1 tsp of vanilla extract

1 tsp of vanilla, ground

¼ cup of fresh raspberries

½ cup of fresh strawberries

¼ tsp of cinnamon, ground

Preparation:

Combine milk and water in a deep pot. bring it to a boil on a low temperature. Add vanilla and vanilla extract. Stir well and let it boil for about a minute. Remove from the heat and allow it to cool.

Combine milk mixture with all other ingredients in a blender. Blend until smooth and transfer to a serving. Refrigerate for 1 hour before serving.

Nutrition information per serving: Kcal: 79, Protein: 4.6g, Carbs: 10.2g, Fats: 1.6g

24. Sweet Swedish Salmon

Ingredients:

2 medium-sized salmon fillets, boneless

1 tsp of cumin, ground

1 tbsp of olive oil

1 tsp of lime juice

1 tsp of cinnamon, ground

1 tsp of paprika, ground

½ tsp salt

¼ tsp of black pepper, ground

Preparation:

Preheat the oven to 350°F.

Combine lime juice, cinnamon, paprika, salt, and pepper in a mixing bowl.

Place the salmon into the mixture and coat well. Cover with plastic wrap and place in the fridge. Marinade for 30 minutes in the refrigerator.

Now place the salmon pieces onto a greased baking tray. Bake for nearly 6-8 minutes and serve hot.

Nutrition information per serving: Kcal: 117, Protein: 18.2g, Carbs: 12.6g, Fats: 8.3g

25.   Mexi-Pulled Beef

Ingredients:

3 lbs lean beef roast

½ cup apple cider vinegar

1 tbsp of vegetable oil

1 tsp of salt

2 tbsp of dried onions, chopped

1 tbsp of cumin, ground

3 tbsp of onion powder

1 garlic clove, minced

3 tbsp of chili powder

Preparation:

Combine cumin, onion, garlic, chili, and salt in a mixing bowl. Set aside to allow flavors to mingle.

With a cooker's lid off, preheat the oil over a medium-high temperature. Add onions and stir-fry for 5 minutes.

Meanwhile coat and rub the meat with the mixture of spices. Place the beef roast in the cooker and cook for about 10-12 minutes, or until browned.

Now add the remaining ingredients and securely lock the pressure cooker's lid. Set for 8 minutes on high.

Perform a quick release to release the cooker's pressure.

Nutrition information per serving: Kcal: 135, Protein: 15.62g, Carbs: 5.4g, Fats: 8.3g

26.   Fresh Frisee with Walnuts

Ingredients:

1 lb of frisee lettuce, trimmed and roughly torn

¼ cup of walnuts

1 small Honeycrisp apple, cored

¼ cup of champagne vinegar

3 tsp of yellow mustard

½ cup of extra-virgin olive oil

¼ tsp of salt

¼ tsp of black pepper, ground

Preparation:

Combine champagne vinegar, mustard, olive oil, salt, and pepper in a blender. Blend well to combine. Set aside.

Trim and roughly torn the frisee in a bowl. Slice the apple into thin matchsticks. Stir in the walnut and drizzle with blended mixture. Toss well to combine. Serve cold.

Nutrition information per serving: Kcal: 315, Protein: 2.7g, Carbs: 12.3g, Fats: 30.3g

27.   Shrimp Skewers Salad with Lemon Chili Dressing

Ingredients:

For the grilled shrimps and tomatoes:

5 large shrimps, peeled and deveined

8 oz grape tomatoes

1 tbsp of olive oil

2 garlic cloves, crushed

1 tsp of fresh cilantro, minced

½ tsp of turmeric, ground

1 tsp of salt

¼ tsp of black pepper, ground

2 skewers, soaked in water

For the salad:

½ head butter lettuce, roughly chopped

½ medium-sized avocado, pitted, peeled and sliced

For the dressing:

¼ cup of lemon juice, freshly squeezed

¼ cup of extra-virgin olive oil

1 tsp of yellow mustard

¼ tsp of chili powder

½ tsp of cumin, ground

1 tbsp of scallions, minced

¼ tsp of sea salt

Preparation:

Preheat an electric grill over a high temperature. Mix together 3 tablespoons of olive oil, crushed garlic, fresh cilantro, turmeric powder, salt, and pepper. Stir until completely combined.

Skewer shrimps and tomatoes and spread the marinade over it using a kitchen brush. Grill for about 2-3 minutes on each side. Remove from the grill and set aside.

Combine the dressing ingredients in a small bowl. Place the butter lettuce and avocado in a bowl. Top with shrimps and tomatoes, and drizzle with the lemon-chili dressing. Enjoy!

Nutrition information per serving: Kcal: 223, Protein: 3.1g, Carbs: 7.2g, Fats: 21.6g

28. Tuna Steaks with Coriander and Lemon Juice

Ingredients:

¼ cup of fresh coriander, chopped

3 garlic cloves, minced

2 tbsp of lemon juice

½ cup olive oil

4 tuna steaks

½ tsp smoked paprika

½ tsp of cumin, ground

½ tsp of chili powder

½ tsp of salt

¼ tsp of black pepper, ground

Preparation:

Add the coriander, garlic, paprika, cumin, chilli powder and lemon juice in a food processor and pulse to combine. Gradually add in the oil and mix the ingredients until a smooth mixture.

Transfer the mixture into a bowl, add the fish and gently toss to coat the fish evenly with sauce. Chill for at least 2 hours to allow the flavors to penetrate into the fish.

Remove the fish from the chiller and preheat the grill. Lightly brush the grid with oil, place the fish and grill for about 3 to 4 minutes on each side.

Remove the fish from the grill, transfer to a serving plate and serve with lemon wedges or some vegetables.

Nutrition information per serving: Kcal: 513, Protein: 54.6g, Carbs: 1.2g, Fats: 31.7g

29.   Fresh Cabbage Lamb Stew

Ingredients:

3 lbs of lamb, boneless, pre-cooked

1 ½ lbs of fresh cabbage

1 large red onion, peeled and sliced

4 garlic cloves, crushed

1 large tomato, finely chopped

½ cup of parsley, finely chopped

4 tbsp of extra-virgin olive oil

6 cups of water

3 bay leaves

Preparation:

Pour 6 cups of water into the pressure pot and add the meat. Securely lock the cooker's lid and set for 10 minutes on high.

Perform a quick release to release the cooker's pressure.

Now add the vegetables and spices. Pour enough water to cover all ingredients. Securely lock the cooker's lid again and set for 25 minutes on high.

Serve warm.

Nutrition information per serving: Kcal: 401, Protein: 31.86g, Carbs: 62.13g, Fats: 5.12g

30.   Blueberry Honey Smoothie

Ingredients:

1 cup of fresh blueberries

¼ cup of almonds, toasted

1 tbsp of chia seeds

1 cup of almond milk

2 tbsp of honey, raw

A handful of ice cubes

Preparation:

Combine all ingredients in a blender. Blend until smooth and transfer to a serving glasses. Serve immediately.

Nutrition information per serving: Kcal: 225, Protein: 11.4g, Carbs: 31.3g, Fats: 8.1g

31. Chicken Honey with Spring Onions

Ingredients:

1 lb of chicken thighs, cut into bite-sized pieces

4 tbsp of honey, raw

6 spring onions, chopped

1 tbsp of fresh mint, finely chopped

6 tsp of cinnamon, ground

1 tbsp of coconut oil

1 tsp of cumin, ground

1 tsp of black pepper, ground

1 tsp of sea salt

Preparation:

Preheat the oil in a large nonstick saucepan over a medium-sized temperature. Add meat and cook for about 8-10 minutes, or until golden brown.

Add chopped onion and toss for another 3 minutes. Add the seasoning and the cumin to it. Sprinkle the cinnamon and add the honey. Toss for 5 minutes more and check if the chicken has cooked through.

Garnish with mint and serve hot.

Nutrition information per serving: Kcal: 105, Protein: 12.9g, Carbs: 11.8g, Fats: 1.1g

32. Fresh Coriander Soup

Ingredients:

4 cups of vegetable broth

2 green chili pepper, finely chopped

6 medium-sized tomatoes, halved

½ tsp of cumin, ground

1 red onion chopped

2 cups of fresh coriander, chopped

1 tsp of almond flour

¼ cup of fresh parsley, chopped

2 tbsp of ginger garlic paste

½ tsp of coriander, chopped

½ tsp of black pepper, ground

½ tsp of sea salt

1 tsp of almond butter

Preparation:

In a large pot, melt the almond butter and fry the chopped red onion for nearly 3 minutes. Add the ginger garlic paste to it.

Add the pepper, salt, coriander, cumin, and green chilies. Toss for 3 minutes and then add the tomatoes. Give it a good stir and then pour in the broth.

Cook on low heat for about 1 hour. Serve hot.

Nutrition information per serving: Kcal: 115, Protein: 4.2g, Carbs: 18.6g, Fats: 5.3g

33.   Roasted Lamb Chops

Ingredients:

2x 1 ½ inch-thick lamb loin chops

1 cup of vegetable oil

3 garlic cloves, crushed

1 tbsp of fresh thyme leaves, crushed

1 tbsp of fresh rosemary, crushed

1 tbsp of red pepper, ground

1 tsp of sea salt

Preparation:

Preheat the oven to 350°F.

Combine the oil with crushed garlic, thyme, rosemary, red pepper, and salt. Mix well in a large bowl. Add lamb loin chops and turn to coat. Let it stand in the refrigerator for about 2 hours.

Place the lamb chops in a large, ovenproof skillet. Add 4 tablespoons of marinade and reduce the heat to 300°F. Cook for about 15 minutes and remove from the oven.

Now add remaining marinade, turn over the chops, and cook for 15 more minutes.

Remove from the oven and serve with fresh vegetables. Enjoy!

Nutrition information per serving: Calories: 411, Protein: 45.6g Carbs: 19.4g Fats: 21.2g

34.   German Stew

Ingredients:

3 lbs of beef chuck shoulder, boneless

1 lb of beef marrow bones

1 large carrot, sliced

3 small onions, peeled

1 lb of button mushrooms, sliced

2 cups of beef stock

10 garlic cloves

2 tbsp of olive oil

1 tbsp of dry rosemary, ground

½ tsp of salt

¼ tsp of black pepper, ground

Preparation:

Preheat the oil in a frying skillet over a medium-high temperature. Add beef and brown on both sides. Remove from the skillet and season generously with salt and pepper.

Transfer to a pressure cooker. Add beef bones, sliced carrot, mushrooms, garlic, rosemary and beef stock.

Securely lock the lid and set to 24 minutes on high.

Perform a quick release to release the cooker's pressure. Remove the bones and serve.

Nutrition information per serving: Kcal: 370, Protein: 46.5g, Carbs: 40.2g, Fats: 29.6g

35.   Sweet Corn Salad

Ingredients:

½ cup of Romaine lettuce, finely chopped

½ cup of sweet corn

1 medium-sized red bell pepper, sliced

½ medium-sized green bell pepper, sliced

5 cherry tomatoes, halved

½ red onion, peeled and sliced

1 tsp of dry rosemary, crushed

1 tsp of lime juice

Preparation:

Wash and cut the bell peppers in half. Remove the seeds and the pulp. Slice into thin slices.

Peel and slice the onion.

Use a big serving platter and arrange the vegetables. You can play with some colors, or even add some ingredients you like. Sprinkle with some rosemary and fresh lime juice. Serve immediately.

Nutrition information per serving: Kcal: 370, Protein: 46.5g, Carbs: 40.2g, Fats: 29.6g

36.   Healthy Leek Stew

Ingredients:

6 large leeks, trimmed

1 lb of lean beef

1 bay leaf

1 medium-sized carrot, sliced

¼ cup of celery, chopped

1 small onion, peeled and sliced

¼ tsp of black pepper, ground

½ tsp of salt

5 tbsp of extra-virgin olive oil

½ tsp of dry rosemary, finely chopped

Preparation:

Grease the bottom of the pressure cooker with 2 tablespoons of olive oil. Coat the meat with some salt and pepper and place in the cooking pot.

Add sliced onion, carrot, celery, and 1 bay leaf. Pour enough water to cover all ingredients and seal the lid. Bring the cooker up to full pressure and reduce to a minimum. Cook for 45 minutes. Remove from the heat and set aside.

Trim the leeks and remove the first two layers. Chop into bite-sized pieces. Heat up the olive oil over medium-high temperature and stir-fry the leeks for several minutes.

Remove the meat from the cooking pot. Chop into smaller pieces and add to the frying skillet. Add dry rosemary and some salt to taste. Cook for another 10-12 minutes.

Nutrition information per serving: Kcal: 420, Protein: 19.3g, Carbs: 25.5g, Fats: 27.4g

37.   Coconut Pudding

Ingredients:

2 cups of coconut milk

1 tbsp of walnuts, finely chopped

1 tbsp of hazelnuts, finely chopped

2 tsp of cocoa powder, raw

1 tsp of cinnamon, ground

½ tbsp of vanilla powder

1 tsp of honey

Preparation:

Pour 2 cups of milk into a deep pot and bring it to a boil.

Add nuts, cocoa, honey, vanilla, and stir well. Cook for about 10 minutes, or until you get a creamy mixture.

Stir in some cinnamon and remove from the heat. Allow it to cool in the refrigerator before serving.

Nutrition information per serving: Kcal: 140, Protein: 3.4g, Carbs: 20.6, Fats: 4.6g

38. Italian Casserole

Ingredients:

4 large eggplants, sliced

2 medium-sized onions, peeled and chopped

10 large tomatoes, roughly chopped

7 oz green olives

7 oz capers

1 medium-sized chili pepper

2 stalks of celery, chopped

½ cup of extra-virgin olive oil

3 tbsp of apple cider vinegar

1 tsp of salt

1 tsp of honey

½ tbsp of basil, dry

Preparation:

Chop the eggplants into bite-sized pieces and season with some salt. Allow it to stand for about 30 minutes and rinse well.

Transfer to a crock pot and add other ingredients. Cover and cook for about 2 hours over a medium temperature.

It can stand in the refrigerator for a couple of days.

Nutrition information per serving: Kcal: 98, Protein: 12.3g, Carbs: 19.4g, Fats: 9.6g

39.   Baby Spinach & Apple Smoothie

Ingredients:

½ medium-sized apple, peeled and sliced

1 cup of baby spinach, finely chopped

1 cup of orange juice, freshly squeezed

2 tbsp of flaxseeds

1 tsp of honey, raw

Preparation:

Combine all ingredients except ice cubes in a blender; purée until smooth. Add ice cubes and re-blend. Transfer the mixture to serving glasses. Enjoy!

Nutrition information per serving: Kcal: 140, Protein: 7.5g, Carbs: 24.0g, Fats: 2.4g

40.   Creamy Broccoli Soup with Lemon Juice

Ingredients:

2 oz of fresh broccoli, trimmed

¼ cup of fresh parsley, finely chopped

1 tsp of dried thyme, ground

1 tbsp of fresh lemon juice

¼ tsp of chili pepper, ground

3 tbsp of olive oil

1 tbsp of cashew cream

Preparation:

Place the broccoli in a deep pot and pour enough water to cover. Bring it to a boil and cook until tender. Remove from the heat and drain.

Transfer to a food processor. Add fresh parsley, thyme, and about ½ cup of water. Pulse until smooth mixture. Return to a pot and add some more water. Bring it to a boil and reduce the temperature to low. Cook for 10 minutes.

Stir in some olive oil and cashew cream, sprinkle with ground chili pepper and add fresh lemon juice. Serve warm.

Nutrition information per serving: Kcal: 72, Protein: 12.4g, Carbs: 15.8g, Fats: 8.3g

41.   Wild Salmon with Fresh Dill

Ingredients:

1 lb of wild salmon, thinly sliced

½ cup of lemon juice, freshly squeezed

1 garlic clove, crushed

1 large egg, beaten

½ tsp of sea salt

1 tbsp of dry parsley, crushed

½ cup of fresh dill, chopped

¼ cup of extra virgin olive oil

2 tbsp of olive oil

Preparation:

Preheat the oven to 350°F.

Combine the olive oil with lemon juice, crushed garlic clove, one egg, salt, and parsley. Mix well and place the salmon slices in it. Cover and marinate for about an hour.

Pour the salmon slices along with marinade in a small baking dish. Bake for 35 minutes. Remove from the oven, and sprinkle with fresh mint.

Nutrition information per serving: Kcal: 235, Protein: 27.3g, Carbs: 5.8, Fats: 9.2g

42.   Cider Mustard Chicken Breast

Ingredients:

2 chicken breasts, boneless and skinless

¼ cup of apple cider vinegar

¼ cup of extra-virgin olive oil

2 garlic cloves, crushed

2 tbsp of yellow mustard

½ tsp of green pepper, freshly ground

2 tbsp of olive oil

Preparation:

Wash and pat dry meat. Place it on a cutting board and season with ground green pepper.

In a large bowl, combine the apple vinegar, olive oil, garlic and mustard to make a marinade. Soak the chicken breast into this marinade and make sure it all gets coated nicely. Cover and place in the refrigerator for at least 2 hours (the best option is to keep it in the refrigerator overnight).

Preheat 1 tablespoon of oil in a large skillet over a medium-high temperature. Add chicken and fry for 7-10 minutes on each side, until nice crispy and light brown. Add some of the marinade mixture while frying the chicken. These juices will make the meat soft. Stir occasionally and check if the chicken is fully cooked. Serve.

Nutrition information per serving: Kcal: 396, Protein: 33.3g, Carbs: 1.2g, Fats: 28.3g

43.   Northern Pate

Ingredients:

2 salmon filets, skinless and boneless

½ tsp of dry rosemary

1/8 tsp of sea salt

¼ tsp of chili pepper, ground

1 tbsp of fresh lemon juice

1 tbsp of extra-virgin olive oil

Preparation:

Wash and pat dry the salmon fillets. Cut into bite- sized pieces and set aside.

Heat up the olive oil in a large skillet over amedium high temperature. Add tuna chops and cook for about 10 minutes, stirring constantly. Remove from the heat and transfer to a food processor.

Add 2 tablespoons of olive oil, lemon juice, salt, chili pepper and rosemary. Process well until nicely combined. Serve with some fresh vegetables.

Nutrition information per serving: Kcal: 240, Protein: 20.2g, Carbs: 1.2g, Fats: 16.3g

44. Fresh Mint Smoothie

Ingredients:

1 cup of chopped broccoli

¼ cup of spinach, chopped

½ cup of water

½ cup of coconut water, unsweetened

1 tbsp of walnuts, ground

A few mint leaves

Preparation:

Wash the vegetables and place into a blender. Put some ice cubes and blend together until smooth mixture.

Top with walnuts and garnish with mint leaves.

Nutrition information per serving: Kcal: 94, Protein: 4.9g, Carbs: 12g, Fats: 2.7g

45. Almond Butter Chocolate

Ingredients:

8 oz cocoa, raw

1 cup of almond butter, melted

1 cup of almond milk

¼ cup of almond flour

4 large eggs

1 cup of honey, raw

5 tbsp of almond cream

Preparation:

Preheat the oven to 300°F.

Place some baking paper over a baking dish and set aside.

Combine all dry ingredients in a large bowl and mix well to combine. Whisk in the eggs, melted almond butter, almond milk, and almond cream.

Transfer the mixture to a prepared baking dish and bake for about 30-35 minutes. Allow it to cool for 1 hour and serve.

Nutrition information per serving: Kcal: 212, Protein: 1.6g, Carbs: 31.3, Fats: 11.4g

46.　Sweet Chicken Thighs

Ingredients:

2 lbs of chicken thighs, boneless

2 medium-sized onions, chopped

2 small chili peppers, chopped

1 cup of chicken broth

¼ cup of fresh orange juice

1 tsp of organic orange extract

2 tbsp of extra-virgin olive oil

1 tsp of barbeque seasoning mix

1 small red onion, chopped

Preparation:

Preheat the oven to 350°F.

Heat up the olive oil in a large saucepan over a medium-high temperature. Add chopped onions and stir-fry for several minutes, until golden color.

Combine chili peppers, orange juice and orange extract in a food processor. Blend for 30 seconds. Add this mixture to a saucepan and stir well. Reduce heat to simmer.

Coat the chicken with barbecue seasoning mix and put it into a saucepan. Add chicken broth and bring it to a boil. Cook over a medium-high temperature until all the water evaporates. Remove from the heat.

Place the chicken into a large baking dish. Bake for about 15 minutes to get a nice crispy, golden brown color.

Nutrition information per serving: Kcal: 170, Protein: 38.5g, Carbs: 11.6g, Fats: 21.7g

47.   Vanilla Mousse

Ingredients:

½ cup of blueberries

¼ cup of strawberries

½ glass of coconut milk

2 cups of water

1 tbsp of almond cream

1 tbsp of powdered vanilla

½ tsp of cinnamon

Preparation:

Combine the ingredients in a food processor and pulse until you get a nice smooth mixture. Top with mixed nuts or seeds on your choice.

Nutrition information per serving: Kcal: 134 Protein: 11.3g, Carbs: 38.3, Fats: 15.9g

48.   Cashew Cream and Avocado Puree

Ingredients:

2 large eggs

2 egg whites

1 tbsp of cashew cream

½ cup of almond milk

1 ripe avocado, pitted, peeled, and roughly chopped

1 tbsp of fresh mint leaves, finely chopped

1 tsp of salt

Preparation:

Hard boil the eggs for about 8-10 minutes. Remove from the heat and allow it to cool.

Peel and cut the eggs. Mash with a fork. Separate the egg whites from yolks.

Peel and chop avocado. Place it in a blender. Add almond milk, eggs, egg whites, cashew cream, salt, and mint leaves.

Blend well for about 30 seconds. Serve cold.

Nutrition information per serving: Kcal: 187, Protein: 12.8g, Carbs: 7.4g, Fats: 4.5g

49.   Grilled Chicken Breast with Parsley

Ingredients:

1 large chicken breasts, skinless and boneless, chopped

¼ cup of extra virgin olive oil

3 garlic cloves, crushed

½ cup of fresh parsley, chopped

1 tbsp of fresh lime juice

1 tsp of salt

Preparation:

Combine the olive oil with crushed garlic cloves, finely chopped parsley, fresh lime juice and some salt.

Wash and pat dry the meat and cut into 1-inch thick pieces. Pour the olive oil mixture over the meat and let it stand for about 15 minutes.

Preheat the grill pan over a medium-high temperature. Add 2 tablespoons of marinade in the grill pan and chicken fillets. Cook for about 15 minutes.

Remove from the pan and serve with some vegetables of your choice.

Nutrition information per serving: Kcal: 439, Protein: 44.2g, Carbs: 1.6g, Fats: 28.1g

50.   Ginger Smoothie

Ingredients:

1 cup of mixed blueberries, raspberries, blackberries and strawberries

½ cup of baby spinach, chopped

½ cup of coconut milk

1 ½ cup of water

¼ tsp of ginger, ground

A handful of fresh mint leaves

Preparation:

Wash the baby spinach and combine with other ingredients in a blender. Mix well for 30 seconds. Serve immediately.

Nutrition information per serving: Kcal: 72, Protein: 6.4g, Carbs: 11.3g, Fats: 2.9g

51.   Lean Beef and Mangel Stew

Ingredients:

7 oz of lean beef

1 large red onion, chopped

4 tbsp of olive oil

½ chili pepper, sliced

3 cups of water

8 oz of mangel, diced

2 medium -sized sweet potatoes, chopped

3 oz of broccoli, trimmed

1 large carrot, chopped

1 large tomato, sliced in cubes

½ cup of tomato sauce

8 cups of water

¼ tsp of Cayenne pepper

2 tbsp of all-purpose flour

Preparation:

Preheat 2 tablespoons of oil in a pot over a medium-high temperature. Add chopped onion and fry for a few minutes, or until golden brown.

Now, add the lean beef, 4 cups of water, and a pinch of salt. Cover and leave it to cook for 15 minutes.

Remove from the heat and add prepared vegetables and tomato sauce. Add 4 more cups of water and transfer to a slow cooker.

Meanwhile, heat up the remaining oil over a medium-high temperature. Add cayenne pepper and flour and stir well. Add the mixture to the slow cooker and cook for about 2 hours. Remove from the heat and give it a good stir before serving.

Nutrition information per serving: Kcal: 295, Protein: 35.4g Carbs: 39.5g Fats: 19.3g

52. Cilantro Pork Stew

Ingredients:

8 oz of pork shoulder, cut into 1-inch thick pieces

1 small onion, sliced

1 cup of beef stock

¼ cup of water

½ cup of green tomatillo salsa

A handful of fresh cilantro, roughly chopped

1 tsp of salt

¼ tsp of black pepper, ground

Preparation:

Place the meat in a large glass bowl. Coat well with salt and pepper.

Place the meat and sliced onion in a deep pot. Pour the beef stock and bring it to a boil. Reduce the heat and add about ½ cup of water and green tomatillo salsa.

Mix well, cover and simmer for about 40 minutes, stirring occasionally.

Serve with fresh cilantro.

Nutrition information per serving: Kcal: 274 Protein: 27.3g, Carbs: 21.1g, Fats: 8.5g

53.   Grilled Trout with Smoked Paprika

Ingredients:

7 oz of fresh trout, cleaned

¼ cup of fresh coriander, chopped

2 garlic cloves, crushed

¼ cup of lemon juice

½ tsp smoked paprika

½ tsp cumin, ground

½ tsp chili powder

¼ tsp of black pepper, ground

¼ cup of extra-virgin olive oil

Preparation:

Combine coriander, crushed garlic, paprika, cumin, chili powder, lemon juice, and olive oil in a food processor and pulse to combine.

Transfer the mixture into a bowl,and then add the fish. Gently toss to coat the fish evenly with sauce. Chill for at least 1 hour to allow the flavor to penetrate into the fish.

Remove the fish from the refrigerator and preheat the grill pan. Place the fish and grill for about 3-4 minutes on each side.

Remove the fish from the grill, transfer to a serving plate and serve with lemon or some vegetables of your choice.

Nutrition information per serving: Kcal: 143, Protein: 21.8g, Carbs: 0.6g, Fats: 8.9g

ADDITIONAL TITLES FROM THIS AUTHOR

70 Effective Meal Recipes to Prevent and Solve Being Overweight: Burn Fat Fast by Using Proper Dieting and Smart Nutrition

By

Joe Correa CSN

48 Acne Solving Meal Recipes: The Fast and Natural Path to Fixing Your Acne Problems in Less Than 10 Days!

By

Joe Correa CSN

41 Alzheimer's Preventing Meal Recipes: Reduce or Eliminate Your Alzheimer's Condition in 30 Days or Less!

By

Joe Correa CSN

70 Effective Breast Cancer Meal Recipes: Prevent and Fight Breast Cancer with Smart Nutrition and Powerful Foods

By

Joe Correa CSN

www.ingramcontent.com/pod-product-compliance
Lightning Source LLC
Chambersburg PA
CBHW051030030426
42336CB00015B/2808